Revitalize Your Health

Intermittent Fasting for Women Over 40

Samantha Jameson

All rights reserved. No part of this publication may be reproduced, distributed, or transmitted in any form or by any means, including photocopying, recording, or other electronic or mechanical methods, without the prior written permission of the publisher, except in the case of brief quotations embodied in critical reviews and certain other noncommercial uses permitted by copyright law.

Copyright © Samantha Jameson , 2023.

Table of Contents

- The Power of Intermittent Fasting for Women Over 40

Introduction

Purpose of the Book

Mrs. Ian was a middle-aged woman in her early 40s who was always struggling with her weight. She was tired of trying out different diets and exercising regimes that never seemed to work for her. One day, she stumbled upon Intermittent Fasting (IF) and decided to give it a try.

At first, Mrs. Ian was skeptical about IF, but after reading several articles and researching the benefits, she decided to give it a chance. She started with a 16/8 method where she would fast for 16 hours and eat within an 8-hour window. She noticed a significant change in her body within the first two weeks of starting IF.

The most remarkable change that Mrs. Ian noticed was that she was able to control her cravings better and was eating smaller portions. She found that she was no longer snacking on junk food and was eating healthier meals. Her energy levels also increased, and she felt more focused throughout the day.

One of the most significant benefits that Mrs. Ian noticed was that she was able to lose weight in a healthy and sustainable way. She found that she was not only losing weight, but she was also building muscle, which was something she had struggled with for years.

However, Mrs. Ian did face some challenges when starting IF. She found that the first few days were tough, and she was feeling a bit lethargic and sluggish. But as she continued with IF, she found that her body was adjusting, and she was no longer feeling fatigued.

In conclusion, Mrs. Ian is grateful that she discovered Intermittent Fasting and how it has changed her life. She no longer struggles with her weight, and she feels healthier and more energetic than ever before. She would highly recommend Intermittent Fasting to any woman over 40 who is looking to live a healthier life.

The purpose of the book 'Revitalize Your Health: Intermittent Fasting for Women Over 40' is to educate and inform women over the age of 40 about the health benefits of intermittent fasting and how to implement it into their daily lives. The book focuses on the specific challenges faced by women in this age group and provides customized advice and guidance on how to overcome them. The book covers topics such as the science behind intermittent fasting, how to get started, common myths and misconceptions, how to overcome challenges, and how to incorporate it into a busy lifestyle. The book aims to help women improve their health, boost their energy levels, and reduce their risk of chronic diseases. Through its comprehensive approach, the book provides a roadmap for women to take control of their health and improve their overall well-being.

Benefits of Intermittent Fasting for Women Over 40

For women over 40, intermittent fasting may offer the following advantages:

Weight reduction: By lowering total calorie intake and encouraging fat loss, intermittent fasting may aid in weight loss.

Intermittent fasting may assist to increase insulin sensitivity, which can help to control blood sugar levels and lower the risk of type 2 diabetes.

Increased energy: Intermittent fasting may boost mental acuity and energy levels.

Reduced inflammation: Intermittent fasting has been shown to be effective in reducing inflammation, which has been linked to a number of chronic conditions, such as arthritis and heart disease.

Better heart health: Studies have indicated that intermittent fasting lowers blood pressure and lowers levels of harmful cholesterol.

Intermittent fasting has been linked to a longer lifespan and a lower chance of developing age-related disorders.

It is important to note that individual outcomes may differ and that not all women may react to intermittent fasting similarly. A doctor should be consulted before beginning an intermittent fasting strategy.

Understanding Intermittent Fasting

A practice of eating called intermittent fasting (IF) alternates between periods of fasting and eating. As it does not forbid any particular foods or macronutrients, it is not a diet in the conventional sense. Instead of what you eat, the emphasis is on when you eat.

IF comes in a variety of forms, including:

The practice of time-restricted feeding (TRF) is limiting daily food consumption to a certain window of time, such as 12–16 hours of eating and 12–20 hours of fasting.
Alternate-day fasting entails eating normally one day and severely limiting calorie intake the next day.
The 5:2 diet calls for eating normally five days a week while limiting caloric intake to 500–600 calories the other two.
IF may be modified to fit unique demands and objectives. It's crucial to remember that

women over 40 may have different nutritional needs, and their IF strategy may need to be adjusted as a result. Before beginning an IF plan, women over 40 with a history of disordered eating should also speak with a doctor or dietitian.

To guarantee proper nutrition, it's crucial to drink plenty of water when fasting and eat meals high in nutrients while eating. It's also advised that you pay attention to your body and modify your IF strategy as necessary.

To sum up, intermittent fasting is an eating pattern that alternates between times of fasting and eating and may be tailored to a person's specific requirements. Before beginning an IF strategy, women over 40 should speak with a medical expert since they could have distinct needs.

Chapter 1

The Science of Intermittent Fasting

How Intermittent Fasting Works

Over the years, intermittent fasting has become more and more well-liked as a diet strategy, particularly among women over 40. This eating pattern, which involves alternating between eating and fasting, is considered to have a number of positive health effects. The idea behind intermittent fasting is that it strengthens the immune system, enhances metabolism, and improves insulin sensitivity. This sort of diet may assist women over 40 who are nearing menopause since it can help to manage the hormonal swings that take place during this period.

The body is placed into a condition of caloric restriction, which is the basic mechanism by which intermittent fasting functions. This deprives the body of energy, which causes the production of growth hormone and encourages the metabolism to speed up. This results in a rise in insulin sensitivity and a decrease in body fat as a result. Fasting is also thought to strengthen the immune system, lower oxidative stress and inflammation, and enhance general health.

Hormone regulation is one of the key advantages of intermittent fasting for women over 40. Women who are going through menopause notice a drop in estrogen levels, which may cause a variety of symptoms including hot flashes, mood changes, and weight gain. By lowering insulin resistance and encouraging the generation of growth hormone, intermittent fasting may assist to regulate hormones. In turn, this promotes better hormonal balance all around and menstrual cycle regulation.

Intermittent fasting may enhance metabolism in addition to hormone regulation. This is due to the fact that when the body is under a calorie limitation, it is compelled to burn fat that has been stored as fuel, which raises metabolism. This kind of diet may also aid in lowering the chance of developing metabolic diseases, which are frequent in women over 40 and include type 2 diabetes and obesity.

A good effect on mental health is also possible with intermittent fasting. According to studies, this kind of diet may enhance mood and cognitive performance while lowering levels of stress and anxiety. This is due to the fact that fasting has been found to enhance the synthesis of BDNF, a protein that is essential for the development and survival of nerve cells.

There are several forms of intermittent fasting, and each has its own unique guidelines and limitations. Alternate-day fasting, in which people eat every other day, and time-restricted fasting, in which people only eat during certain times of the day, are two common approaches. Before beginning any intermittent fasting regimen, women over 40 should speak with a healthcare provider to be sure it is suitable for their particular health requirements.

In conclusion, intermittent fasting is a well-liked and successful diet strategy that may assist women over 40 in a variety of ways. The body is placed into a condition of calorie restriction, which helps to enhance metabolism, regulate hormones, raise insulin sensitivity, and strengthen the immune system. This kind of diet may be beneficial for women who are close to menopause since it can control the hormonal swings that take place during this period. Before beginning any form of intermittent fasting program, it is crucial to speak with a medical practitioner to be sure it is suitable for your particular health requirements.

How it Affects the Body

A practice of eating known as intermittent fasting (IF) alternates between periods of fasting and feasting. It is becoming more and more well-liked as a strategy to encourage weight reduction, enhance general health, and lengthen longevity.

Given that the body's metabolism typically slows down as we get older, IF may be particularly helpful for women over 40. Here are a few ways that IF may benefit a woman's body:

Weight loss: IF may assist with weight reduction and improve body composition by limiting calorie intake during fasting periods. Additionally, this may enhance general health and lower the risk of obesity-related illnesses including diabetes, heart disease, and several types of cancer.

Fasting has been shown to increase insulin sensitivity, which is crucial for women over 40 since they are more prone to developing insulin resistance and type 2 diabetes.

Balance of hormones: Insulin, cortisol, and leptin, which are involved in metabolism, the stress response, and appetite regulation, may all be controlled by fasting. Hormone regulation during IF may aid in weight control since hormonal abnormalities often result in weight gain.

Reduced inflammation: Heart disease, diabetes, and a few types of cancer have all been associated with chronic inflammation. It has been shown that fasting lowers inflammatory indicators in the body, improving general health and lowering the likelihood of developing chronic illnesses.

Improved memory, concentration, and attention have all been related to fasting's positive effects on cognitive performance. Women over 40 who may be suffering age-related decreases in cognitive performance may find this to be of particular importance.

While IF may be beneficial, not everyone should use it, particularly those with specific medical issues, those who are pregnant, or those who are nursing. It's also crucial to pay attention to your body's signals and modify as necessary.

In conclusion, intermittent fasting may benefit a woman's physique beyond the age of 40. IF may enhance general health and lower the risk of chronic illnesses by increasing weight reduction, enhancing insulin sensitivity, regulating hormones, lowering inflammation, and enhancing cognitive function. However, it's crucial to speak with a doctor before beginning any new dietary regimen, particularly for women with certain health problems.

The Different Types of Intermittent Fasting

For women over 40, intermittent fasting has grown in popularity as a means of weight loss and general health improvement. However, there are several forms of intermittent fasting that may accommodate various objectives and lifestyles. Women over 40 will be better able to choose the appropriate strategy for their particular demands if they are aware of these categories.

The most common kind of intermittent fasting, known as the 16/8 Method, calls for a 16-hour fast followed by an 8-hour window for eating. For instance, if your last meal is at 7 p.m., your next meal won't be until 11am the following day. Women who want an easy, adaptable approach to include fasting into their daily schedule will love this strategy.

The 5:2 Diet: This plan calls for eating regularly for five days and then limiting calories to 500–600 for two separate days. This strategy is appropriate for ladies who wish to fast in a more disciplined manner while still regularly indulging in their favorite meals.

The alternate-day fasting entails missing breakfast or limiting calorie intake to 500–600 calories every other day. Women who can adhere to a rigid schedule and are searching for a more active approach to fasting might use this strategy.

The Eat Stop Eat Method calls for a 24-hour fast once or twice every week. For instance, if your last meal is at 7 p.m., your next meal won't be until 7 p.m. the following day. This technique is excellent for ladies who want to fast but may find it challenging to fast for prolonged periods of time.

Time-Restricted Feeding: This entails limiting when you eat each day to a certain window of time, often between 8 and 12 hours. If you began eating at noon, for instance, you wouldn't eat again until eight o'clock. Women who wish to include fasting into their routine but still want to consume a variety of meals throughout the day might use this strategy.

It is crucial to make sure that women over 40 are still obtaining enough nutrients to maintain their general health, regardless of the form of intermittent fasting they select. This may be accomplished by consuming nutrient-dense foods within their eating window, such as fruits, vegetables, lean meats, and whole grains.

Before beginning any new eating plan, it's also advisable to see a healthcare provider, particularly for women over 40 who could already be dealing with health issues. In order to improve health and lose weight, intermittent fasting may be a safe and successful method, but it must be done in a manner that is sustainable and beneficial to overall wellbeing.

As a result, women over 40 have a variety of alternatives for incorporating intermittent fasting into their life. Finding the best strategy to fit unique objectives and lifestyles is crucial, as is making sure enough nutrition is maintained. Women over 40 who want to improve their health and wellness may effectively use intermittent fasting by talking to a healthcare practitioner and carefully weighing their alternatives.

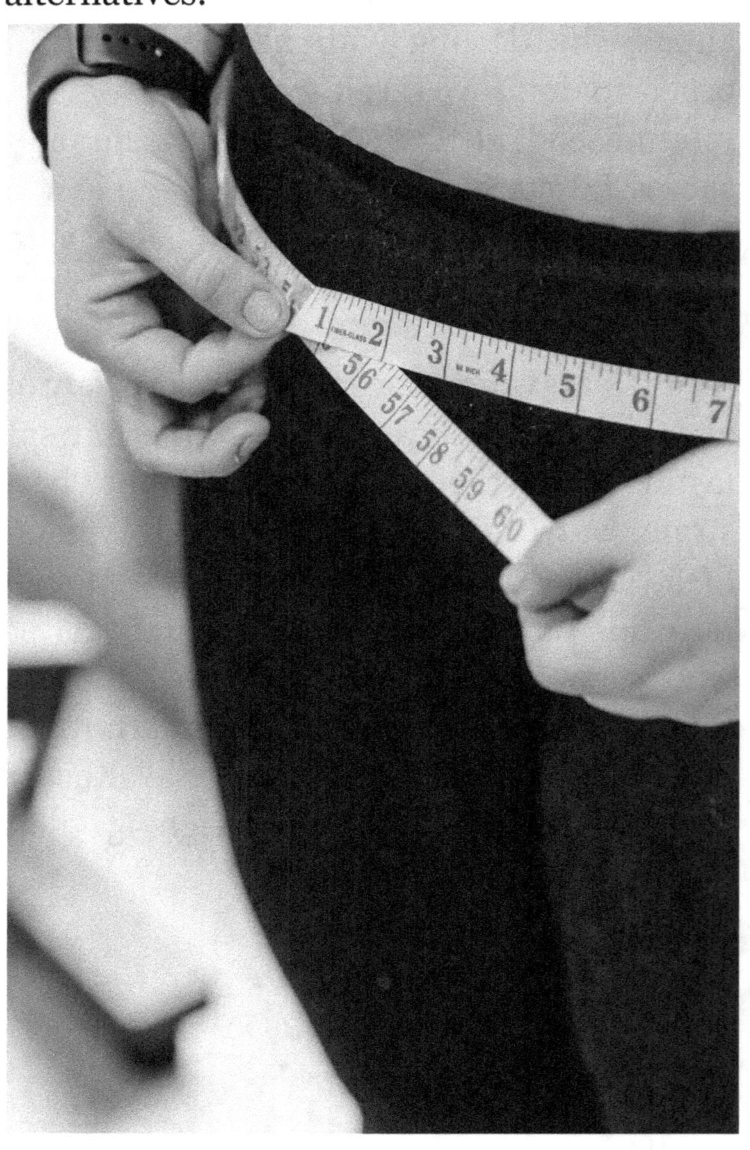

Chapter 2

Getting Started with Intermittent Fasting

Preparing Your Body and Mind

A wonderful choice for women over 40 who are seeking for a new technique to enhance their general health and wellbeing is intermittent fasting, which is a developing trend in the health and wellness industry. It has been shown that intermittent fasting, which comprises periods of fasting followed by intervals of regular eating, offers a variety of advantages, including weight reduction, increased energy, and decreased inflammation. However, it's crucial to make sure you are properly prepared, both physically and emotionally, before beginning any new health program. The following information will help you prepare your body and mind for intermittent fasting.

Physical getting ready

Water consumption is essential during a fast in order to keep your body hydrated and prevent dehydration. Drink water before, during, and after your fast, and aim to consume at least 8 glasses each day.

Gradual Expansion: To give your body time to adapt, gradually extend your fasting intervals. As your body adjusts, go up to longer fasts starting with shorter ones.

Healthy eating: During your mealtimes, be sure to consume a healthy, balanced diet. By doing this, you'll make it easier for your body to get the nutrients it needs to operate normally throughout your fasting intervals.

Exercise: Keeping your body active and energetic might assist to make fasting easier. Exercise is also vital for general health and fitness. Aim to work out for at least 30 minutes each day, and you may want to think about adding HIIT to your regimen.

Mental rehearsing

Make sure you comprehend the advantages of intermittent fasting and how it functions. This will assist you in maintaining your attention and motivation during fasting.

Support: Surround yourself with positive individuals who will uplift and inspire you. It may be a lot simpler and more pleasurable to travel when you have a companion.

Positive attitude: Concentrate on the advantages of fasting, including increased energy, less inflammation, and weight reduction. This will assist you in maintaining your attention and motivation during fasting.

Self-reflection: Consider your motivations for trying intermittent fasting and your desired outcomes. This will support your motivation and attention while you travel.

Women over 40 who want to enhance their general health and wellbeing might consider intermittent fasting, but it's crucial to be completely ready before beginning. You may make sure that you are emotionally and physically prepared for the road ahead by following the above-described procedures. To ensure that you are at ease and in good health during your fasting periods, keep in mind that it is crucial to pay attention to your body and make any required modifications along the way. Intermittent fasting, when done properly, may improve your overall health and fitness and assist you in reaching your objectives..

Setting Your Fasting Schedule

A diet strategy known as intermittent fasting alternates between periods of eating and fasting. It has gained popularity recently as a means of weight loss and general health improvement, particularly among women over 40. However, since each person's body responds differently to fasting, it might be difficult to choose the plan that is ideal for you.

It's critical to comprehend the various forms of intermittent fasting before beginning your fasting schedule. There is the 16/8 approach, which entails a 16-hour fast followed by an 8-hour interval for eating. The 5:2 diet, in which you eat normally for five days and then fast for two, is another well-liked strategy. Alternate-day fasting is another option, in which you alternate between eating regularly and fasting.

It is important to take your lifestyle and eating habits into account when planning your fasting regimen. The 16/8 technique can be more practical for you if you don't have much time to prepare meals due to a hectic schedule. On the other hand, alternate-day fasting can be a better choice if your schedule is more flexible.

Additionally, it's critical to take your age and hormone levels into account, particularly if you're a woman over 40. Women in this age range are more prone to hormonal imbalances, which may have an impact on their appetite and metabolism. Before beginning any fasting diet, you should speak with your doctor if you have any health issues or are on any drugs.

When fasting, it's crucial to prioritize nutrient-dense meals over processed ones. This will make sure that you are still losing weight while obtaining the nutrients your body needs. You should also make sure to drink enough water to stay hydrated and to assist your body remove toxins.

It's common to first experience some hunger during the fasting intervals. Try to divert your attention from eating to engage in other pursuits, such as exercise, meditation, or reading, to assist you overcome this. Having a support system in place, such as a friend or family member who also practices intermittent fasting, may also be beneficial.

It's crucial to be patient and allow yourself time to adapt when starting a new diet or workout regimen. It is vital to keep experimenting with various fasting regimens until you discover the one that works best for you since intermittent fasting may not be effective for everyone. It's crucial to stop and see your doctor if you have any unfavorable side effects, such as extreme appetite or weakness.

In conclusion, creating an intermittent fasting plan is a personal process that should be customized to your unique demands and way of life. Along with your dietary and lifestyle choices, it's crucial to take your age, hormone levels, and any underlying medical issues into account. You may reach your weight reduction and health objectives while still feeling fulfilled by putting an emphasis on nutrient-dense meals and keeping hydrated.

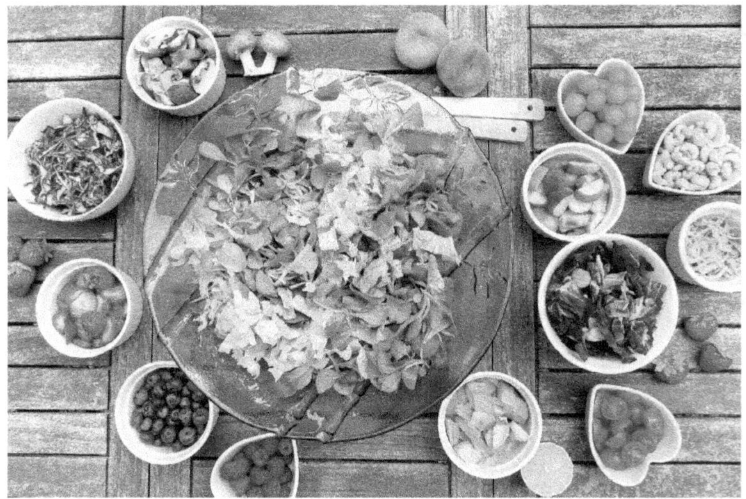

Tips for Success

You could have tried a variety of diets and exercises as a woman over 40 to shed weight and maintain your fitness. The most recent weight reduction fad is intermittent fasting, which may be a fantastic method to get started on your weight loss quest. Here are some pointers for succeeding with IF:

Select the appropriate kind of intermittent fasting: Whole-day fasting, alternate-day fasting, and time-restricted eating are some of the variations. Pick the strategy that works best for you and stay with it. For instance, if you've never fasted before, start by eating just at certain times of the day and then gradually increase the frequency and length of your meals.

Stay hydrated: To keep your body hydrated when fasting, be sure to consume plenty of water. Additionally, water consumption helps lessen symptoms of weariness and hunger.

Plan your meals: When you are intermittently fasting, you must pay attention to the foods you consume throughout your feeding window. Make a nutrition plan in advance and make sure it includes protein, carbs, healthy fats, and fiber.

Exercise regularly: Exercise may increase your metabolism and can help you feel fuller when fasting. At least five days a week, try to get in 30 minutes of moderate-intensity activity, such as walking, cycling, or swimming.

Sleep well: Sleep is important for overall health and may help control your hunger hormones. Try to maintain a regular sleep pattern and aim for at least seven hours of sleep each night.

Remain optimistic: Intermittent fasting may be difficult, so it's important to remain upbeat and goal-focused. Remember your initial motivation for fasting, and surround yourself with encouraging friends and family.

Avoid processed foods: Try to steer clear of processed foods throughout your meal window in favor of whole foods. Processed foods might hinder your attempts to lose weight since they are heavy in calories and lacking in nutrients.

Avoid skipping meals: Women over 40 should avoid skipping meals since they are more likely to develop illnesses like osteoporosis. Make sure to have a balanced meal and refrain from missing meals within your feeding window.

Increase the length and frequency of fasting gradually: Intermittent fasting takes time and patience, therefore it's important to go gently. Don't attempt to push yourself too hard; gradually extend your fasting periods and frequency.

Follow your development: To gauge your progress, keep track of your weight, body measurements, and other indicators of success. Consult your doctor if you develop any negative side effects, such as headaches, lethargy, or vertigo.

In conclusion, women over 40 who want to start losing weight may do so by using intermittent fasting. But it's important to pay attention to what you eat, drink a lot of water, exercise often, get adequate sleep, and have a happy outlook. Keep in mind that losing weight is a process, and success requires patience, perseverance, and time.

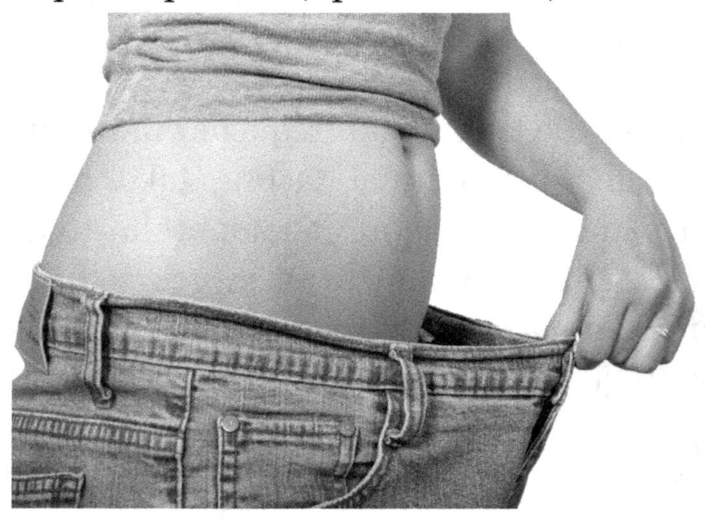

Chapter 3

Making Intermittent Fasting a Lifestyle

Overcoming Challenges

Although intermittent fasting has gained popularity as a weight management and health improvement technique, older women may find it difficult to follow the schedule. Following a rigorous fasting schedule might be challenging for women over 40 because of the many physical and hormonal changes they often experience. In this post, we'll talk about some of the typical difficulties older women who fast intermittently encounter and provide solutions.

One of the most frequent difficulties with intermittent fasting is hunger sensations. The increased hunger that many women over the age of 40 feel during fasting may be brought on by hormonal changes in the body. Women may overcome this by consuming a lot of water, green tea, or herbal tea to curb their appetite. Additionally, they may have low-calorie snacks including fruits, veggies, and nuts.

Dehydration: Dehydration is another difficulty with intermittent fasting. To prevent dehydration, women over 40 should make sure to consume lots of water. Water consumption might also lessen hunger cravings.

Low energy levels may be a side effect of intermittent fasting, particularly at the beginning of the diet. The body could be adapting to the new habit if this happens. By eating a balanced meal within their feeding windows and doing mild exercise, women over 40 may overcome this.

Hormonal Imbalances: For women over 40 who practice intermittent fasting, hormonal imbalances might be a problem. Hormonal imbalances may cause bothersome symptoms including mood swings, irregular menstruation periods, and others. Women may do this by seeing a doctor and thinking about changing their fasting regimen.

Social obligations: For women over 40 who have social responsibilities, intermittent fasting might be difficult. This is due to the fact that food and beverages are often served during social gatherings, which might be enticing while fasting. In order to get around this, ladies should have a small lunch before social gatherings and bring low-calorie snacks.

Maintaining the Schedule: Maintaining the fasting schedule when practicing intermittent fasting calls for commitment and discipline. It may be challenging for busy women over 40 to adhere to a rigid fasting regimen. They may do this by organizing their fasting schedule in advance and adhering to it as much as they can.

In conclusion, by using the advice provided in this article, women over 40 may successfully navigate the difficulties of intermittent fasting. Numerous health advantages may be obtained by intermittent fasting, but it takes commitment and self-control. Before beginning an intermittent fasting diet, women over 40 should also get medical counsel, particularly if they have any health issues. Women over 40 may effectively adhere to an intermittent fasting diet and profit from it with the correct strategy.

Incorporating Exercise and Nutrition

Women over 40 who want to drop a few pounds, boost their general health, and extend their life expectancy are increasingly following the trend of intermittent fasting. Although it is a successful weight-loss method, including exercise and good eating into this regimen may be challenging. However, by adopting the proper strategy, you may maximize the advantages of intermittent fasting and enhance your health and wellbeing.

Two important elements that might have a big influence on the success of your intermittent fasting journey are exercise and diet. Here's how to successfully integrate them.

Exercise:

During intermittent fasting, you set calorie intake restrictions for certain times of the day. This does not, however, imply that you should quit working out. Instead, exercise may help you keep the weight off and increase the overall health advantages of intermittent fasting.

Start with low-impact workouts like stretching, yoga, or walking if you're a novice. You may progressively increase the intensity of your exercises as your body becomes used to the new schedule. It is advised to work out at least 30 minutes each day, three to five times per week.

For women over 40 who desire to speed up their metabolism, high-intensity interval training (HIIT) is a viable choice. Exercises that alternate between high- and low-intensity movements make up HIIT, a quick yet intense workout. It's a fantastic strategy to increase heart rate and burn more calories faster.

Nutrition:

Making sure you consume the proper items throughout your eating window is essential for success with intermittent fasting. Nutrient-dense foods including fruits, vegetables, whole grains, and lean meats must be a part of your diet. These meals will fill you up and provide your body the nourishment it needs to operate correctly.

During your eating window, it's vital to stay away from processed meals and sugary beverages. These meals may negate all the advantages of intermittent fasting since they are heavy in calories and poor in nutrients. To remain hydrated, use herbal teas, water, or green tea.

You are also encouraged to reduce your meal sizes through intermittent fasting. This implies that during your eating window, try to consume smaller, more frequent meals. Eating smaller portions will help you consume fewer calories overall and maintain a healthy weight.

Conclusion:

You may maximize the advantages of intermittent fasting and reach your weight-loss and health objectives by including exercise and nutrition into your daily routine. Make careful to eat nutrient-dense items in your diet as you progressively raise the intensity of your low-impact activities. Don't forget to consume less portions and stay away from processed meals. You may have a better and more meaningful life if you take the appropriate steps.

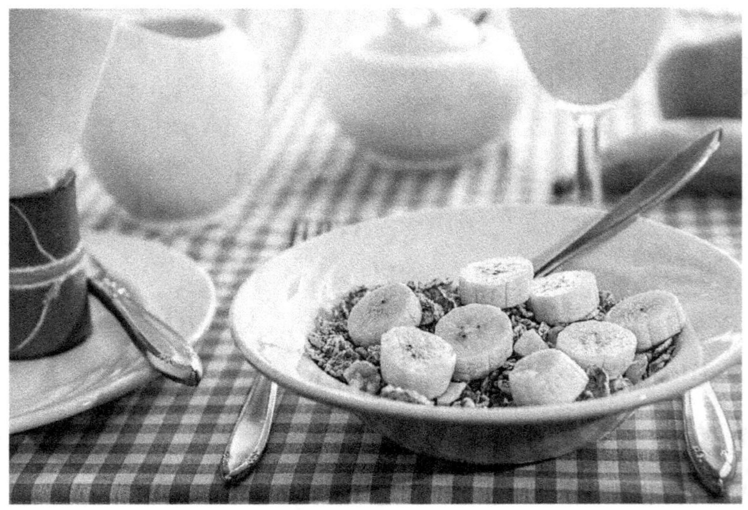

Building a Support System

In recent years, intermittent fasting has gained popularity as a trend among those trying to manage their chronic illnesses, reduce weight, and improve their health. The thought of beginning a new diet or lifestyle change as a woman over 40 might be intimidating, but with the correct support network, it can be a pleasant and life-changing experience.

Creating a support network can keep you motivated, hold you responsible, and provide guidance and encouragement along the road. Finding people who will support your ambitions and be ready to assist you on your path is the first step. This might be a close friend, a member of the family, a work colleague, or even a trained coach or counselor.

It's crucial to find someone you can be open and honest with about your development, difficulties, and successes. It might also be helpful to have a supportive spouse, particularly if they are also thinking about trying intermittent fasting. This may foster a sense of community and provide you someone to rely on when the going gets tough.

There are several online groups and forums devoted particularly to intermittent fasting in addition to one-on-one help. These may be a terrific resource for discovering new dishes, exchanging stories, and getting guidance from others who have experienced something similar to your own. To chronicle your trip and communicate with others, think about joining a Social Media group, taking part in a Personal thread, or even beginning your own blog.

Locating a neighborhood club or organization that focuses on intermittent fasting is another method to create a support network. This may be a terrific method to get in touch with others who are going through similar things, exchange experiences, and pick people's brains. Look for local gatherings, seminars, or courses. To connect with others who share your interests, you may also go to conferences or events devoted to intermittent fasting.

Positivity is one of the most crucial components of creating a support system for intermittent fasting. Even while facing difficulties, surrounding oneself with uplifting, encouraging people may help you stay focused and on course. Try to keep your attention on the advantages of intermittent fasting, such as higher energy, clearer thinking, and better overall health.

Having a support system may also hold you accountable and assist you in staying on course. You are less prone to give in to temptations or stray from your course when you have someone to answer to. Even when you are feeling demotivated, your support network can keep you focused and motivated.

As a woman over 40 beginning an intermittent fasting program, developing a support network is crucial for success. Having a support system, whether it be a personal friend, online community, or local organization, may provide you encouragement, guidance, and accountability. To help you remain motivated and reach your objectives, surround yourself with uplifting, encouraging people and concentrate on the advantages of IF.

Chapter 4

Special Considerations for Women Over 40

Menopause and Intermittent Fasting

The menopause, a biologically normal process, signals the end of a woman's fertile years. It is a stage of transition that starts with a drop in estrogen levels and culminates with the menstrual periods permanently ceasing. Menopause usually occurs in women between the ages of 45 and 55, however others may go through it sooner or later.

A form of diet known as intermittent fasting includes alternating between times of eating and fasting. This eating strategy has been more well-liked recently because of its possible health advantages, which include weight reduction, increased insulin sensitivity, and a decreased chance of developing chronic illnesses. There are numerous methods to practice intermittent fasting, such as limiting calories on certain days of the week or going without food for a predetermined period of time each day.

Intermittent fasting with menopause may have a substantial negative influence on a woman's health and wellbeing. Hot flashes, nocturnal sweats, sleeplessness, and mood swings are just a few of the physical and psychological symptoms of menopause that may result from the drop in estrogen levels. By lowering inflammation and enhancing general health indices, intermittent fasting has been shown to help with some of these symptoms.

Additionally, menopause may raise your chance of developing long-term conditions including heart disease, type 2 diabetes, and obesity. It has been shown that intermittent fasting improves a variety of health indicators, including insulin resistance, oxidative stress, and insulin sensitivity. This may assist to reduce the chance of developing certain illnesses and enhance general health.

Menopausal women over 40 should exercise caution when beginning an intermittent fasting routine, it is crucial to remember. Women at this period of life may be more vulnerable to the side effects of fasting, such as dehydration and vitamin shortages, even though it may be a safe and efficient technique for enhancing health. In addition, menopausal women are more likely to have bone loss, which intermittent fasting may aggravate if not done appropriately.

It is advised that menopausal women interested in attempting intermittent fasting collaborate with a healthcare professional to develop a strategy that is secure and suitable for their particular requirements. This can include keeping an eye on their hormone levels and modifying their fasting regimen as necessary. In order to make sure they are receiving enough of the vital vitamins and minerals they need, women going through menopause should also concentrate on eating nutrient-dense meals and supplementing as necessary.

In conclusion, although menopause and intermittent fasting might be difficult to combine, if done correctly, they can benefit a woman's health and wellbeing. Menopausal women should exercise caution while beginning an intermittent fasting program, although they may benefit from this way of eating with the help of a healthcare professional. Menopausal and intermittent fasting together may benefit women over 40 in several ways, including easing menopause symptoms and lowering their chance of developing chronic illnesses.

Hormonal Changes and Intermittent Fasting

The health and wellbeing of women over 40 are profoundly impacted by hormonal changes and intermittent fasting (IF). Numerous health problems might result from hormonal imbalances brought on by perimenopause and menopause as well as the physiological changes that take place during this period. On the other hand, intermittent fasting is a kind of dieting that alternates between fasting and not fasting. Due to the possible health advantages of this eating strategy, it has become more and more well-liked in recent years. The consequences of hormonal shifts and intermittent fasting on women over 40 will be covered in this article, along with management strategies that may be used to improve general health and wellbeing.

Changes in Hormones in Women Over 40

Hormone production, including that of progesterone and estrogen, decreases in women over 40. Menopause and perimenopause are two hormonal abnormalities that may result from this reduction. A natural transition called menopause occurs when the ovaries cease producing eggs and when less estrogen and progesterone are produced. Numerous symptoms, including hot flashes, nocturnal sweats, mood changes, and exhaustion, may result from this. The transitional stage before menopause, known as perimenopause, may extend for many years. Women may have irregular menstrual cycles, a decline in libido, and other symptoms linked to hormonal imbalances at this period.

Fasting Intermittently and Women Over 40

Fasting and non-fasting phases are alternated throughout an intermittent fasting diet. Due to its potential health advantages, such as weight reduction, increased insulin sensitivity, and decreased inflammation, this kind of dieting has grown in favor. Additionally linked to better mental acuity, less stress levels, and higher-quality sleep is intermittent fasting.

However, because of the hormonal changes they are going through, women over the age of 40 can have different results from intermittent fasting. For instance, the drop in estrogen levels that occurs after menopause might raise the risk of osteoporosis and other illnesses. In older women, intermittent fasting may also have an impact on menstrual cycles and other menstruation-related problems. Additionally, owing to hormonal changes they are going through, women over 40 may feel more stressed while intermittent fasting.

Intermittent fasting and Managing Hormonal Changes for Women Over 40

It's crucial to be aware of the health concerns and get medical counsel before beginning any new dietary plan in order to manage the impact of hormonal changes and intermittent fasting for women over 40.

It is advised that women over 40 concentrate on consuming nutrient-dense meals, such as leafy greens, healthy fats, and lean meats. In order to maintain their general health and wellbeing, kids should also try to consume enough amounts of vitamins and minerals, such as calcium, vitamin D, and iron.

If done safely and mindfully, intermittent fasting may also be advantageous for women over the age of 40. They could decide to fast for 12 hours and eat inside a 12-hour window, for instance. In addition, it is advised that women over 40 pay attention to their bodies and refrain from fasting if they feel weak or exhausted.

Conclusion

Intermittent fasting and hormonal shifts have a big influence on the health and happiness of women over 40. Women over 40 may control these variables and advance general health and wellbeing by concentrating on consuming nutrient-dense meals and being aware of the possible health hazards. It is always important to get medical counsel before beginning any new dietary plan if you have any worries or issues.

Adapting Intermittent Fasting to Your Health Concerns

As a weight reduction and general health technique, intermittent fasting has become more and more popular in recent years. However, it's important to realize that everyone is different, particularly women over 40. What may work for one person may not necessarily work for another. You may accomplish your aims and prevent any unfavorable effects by customizing intermittent fasting to your particular health issues.

A practice of eating called intermittent fasting alternates between periods of fasting and periods of eating. The 16/8 approach, in which you fast for 16 hours and then eat within an 8-hour window, is the most popular one. Other approaches include alternate-day fasting and the 5:2 diet, which allows you to eat normally for five days while limiting your caloric intake to 500–600 calories on the other two.

When implementing intermittent fasting, women over 40 may have certain health issues that need to be taken into consideration. Here are some of the most typical worries and solutions:

Hormonal imbalances: Women going through menopause may have hormonal imbalances that cause mood swings, hot flashes, and weight gain. While prolonged fasting should be avoided since it might worsen hormonal imbalances and raise stress, intermittent fasting can assist in regulating hormones. For women over 40 who are new to fasting, the 16/8 approach is a wonderful place to start.

Bone health: Women over 40 are more susceptible to osteoporosis and should be cautious about placing too strict of a restriction on their calcium consumption. This is due to the fact that calcium is crucial for keeping healthy bones. While intermittent fasting may help increase bone density, it's crucial to make sure you consume enough calcium-rich foods during your eating window, such as dairy products, green leafy vegetables, and tofu.

Low energy: Women over 40 may notice a decline in energy, which makes it challenging to maintain a fasting schedule. In order to prevent this, it's crucial to consume a balanced meal within your eating window and to stay away from items that are heavy in fat and sugar since they might deplete your energy. Also, be sure to get enough sleep, since not getting enough sleep might make you feel more tired.

Digestive problems: Due to hormonal changes and a slowed metabolism, women over 40 may also develop digestive problems, such as bloating and constipation. Eat a balanced diet that includes fiber-rich foods, such as fruits and vegetables, throughout your eating window to prevent these problems. Drinking lots of water is also crucial to maintain proper digestion and to prevent overeating, which may exacerbate digestive problems.

Medication: Women over 40 should exercise caution while adjusting to intermittent fasting if they are taking medication for a medical problem such diabetes, high blood pressure, or heart disease. It's crucial to see your doctor before beginning a fasting routine since fasting may interfere with the treatment of certain medical issues and may change how some drugs are absorbed.

As a result, tailoring intermittent fasting to your unique health challenges may help you accomplish your objectives without experiencing any unfavorable effects. When beginning a fasting routine, women over 40 should take into account their hormones, bone health, energy levels, digestive problems, and medicines. Before beginning any new eating plan, it is always advisable to speak with your doctor to be sure it is healthy for you.

Chapter 5

Meal Planning and Recipes

Planning Your Fasting Days

Day 1:

Breakfast: Green smoothie made with spinach, almond milk, banana, and almond butter.
Lunch: Grilled chicken salad with mixed greens, cherry tomatoes, cucumber, and a lemon vinaigrette.
Dinner: Baked salmon with roasted asparagus and brown rice.

Day 2:

Breakfast: Scrambled eggs with avocado, cherry tomatoes, and whole grain toast.
Lunch: Turkey and cheese wrap with whole grain tortilla, lettuce, and mustard.

Dinner: Grilled shrimp with roasted sweet potatoes and steamed broccoli.

Day 3:

Breakfast: Greek yogurt with berries, chia seeds, and a drizzle of honey.
Lunch: Quinoa salad with roasted vegetables, feta cheese, and a balsamic vinaigrette.
Dinner: Grilled chicken with roasted vegetables and quinoa.

Day 4:

Breakfast: Oatmeal with almond milk, banana, and almond butter.
Lunch: Grilled chicken breast with mixed greens and balsamic vinaigrette.
Dinner: Baked cod with roasted brussels sprouts and brown rice.

Day 5:

Breakfast: Smoothie bowl made with spinach, almond milk, berries, and almond butter.
Lunch: Turkey and cheese sandwich with whole grain bread, lettuce, and mustard.
Dinner: Grilled shrimp with roasted carrots and steamed brown rice.

Day 6:

Breakfast: Scrambled eggs with mushrooms, cherry tomatoes, and whole grain toast.
Lunch: Grilled chicken salad with mixed greens, cherry tomatoes, cucumber, and a lemon vinaigrette.
Dinner: Baked salmon with roasted asparagus and brown rice.

Day 7:

Breakfast: Greek yogurt with berries, chia seeds, and a drizzle of honey.

Lunch: Quinoa salad with roasted vegetables, feta cheese, and a balsamic vinaigrette.

Dinner: Grilled chicken with roasted vegetables and quinoa.

Note: This meal plan is designed for women over 40 who are practicing intermittent fasting and are looking for healthy, nutritious options for their fasting days. It is important to consult with a healthcare provider before starting any new dietary program.

Delicious Recipes for Your Fasting Days

Breakfast Recipes

1. Avocado and eggs on toast

Ingredients:

- 2 slices of whole grain bread
- 1 ripe avocado
- 2 eggs
- Salt and pepper to taste
- Optional: fresh herbs (e.g. cilantro), hot sauce, lemon juice, etc.

Instructions:

- Toast 2 slices of whole grain bread.
- While the bread is toasting, cut 1 ripe avocado in half and remove the pit. Mash the flesh with a fork.
- Fry 2 eggs in a pan over medium heat until the whites are set and the yolks are still runny.
- Spread the mashed avocado over the toasted bread.

- Top with the fried eggs and season with salt and pepper to taste.
- Serve hot and enjoy!

Serving size: 2 slices of toast (1 serving)

Nutritional information per serving:
Calories: approx. 350-400
Protein: 15-18 g
Fat: 26-30 g
Carbohydrates: 20-25 g
Fiber: 8-10 g
Sodium: 300-400 mg (varies based on bread and seasonings used)

Note: Nutritional information may vary based on specific ingredients and serving size.

2. Yogurt with mixed berries and nuts

Ingredients:

- 1 cup Greek yogurt

- 1/2 cup mixed berries (strawberries, raspberries, blueberries, blackberries)
- 1/4 cup chopped nuts (almonds, walnuts, pecans)
- 1 tbsp honey (optional)

Serving Size: 1

Instructions:

- In a bowl, mix the Greek yogurt, mixed berries, chopped nuts, and honey (if using).
- Stir until everything is evenly distributed.
- Serve and enjoy!

Nutritional Value (per serving):

Calories: 300
Total Fat: 20 g
Saturated Fat: 3 g
Cholesterol: 15 mg
Sodium: 130 mg
Total Carbohydrates: 20 g
Dietary Fiber: 4 g

Sugars: 15 g
Protein: 15 g

3. Veggie omelet with mushrooms, tomatoes, and spinach

Ingredients:

- 2 large eggs
- 1/4 cup diced mushrooms
- 1/4 cup diced tomatoes
- 1/4 cup chopped spinach
- Salt and pepper, to taste
- 1 tsp. olive oil

Instructions:

- Heat the olive oil in a medium-sized nonstick skillet over medium heat.
- Add the mushrooms, tomatoes, and spinach and sauté until they are soft, about 3-5 minutes.

- In a separate bowl, whisk together the eggs, salt, and pepper.
- Pour the eggs into the skillet with the vegetables and cook until the bottom is set, about 2 minutes.
- Use a spatula to gently fold the omelet in half and cook until the eggs are set, about 2-3 more minutes.
- Serve immediately.

Nutritional Value (per serving):

Calories: 152
Fat: 11g
Carbohydrates: 4g
Protein: 11g
Fiber: 1g
Serving size: 1 omelet (makes 1 serving)

4. Peanut butter banana smoothie bowl

Ingredients:

- 1 ripe banana

- 1/2 cup unsweetened almond milk
- 1 tablespoon creamy peanut butter
- 1 scoop vanilla protein powder
- 1 teaspoon honey
- 1/4 teaspoon ground cinnamon
- 1/4 teaspoon vanilla extract
- 1/2 cup ice cubes
- Toppings (optional): chopped peanuts, sliced banana, almond butter drizzle

Instructions:

- In a blender, combine the banana, almond milk, peanut butter, protein powder, honey, cinnamon, vanilla extract, and ice cubes.

- Blend until smooth and creamy.

- Pour the smoothie into a bowl and top with your desired toppings.

Serving size: 1 bowl

Nutritional value: (per serving)

Calories: 384
Total Fat: 17g
Saturated Fat: 3g
Trans Fat: 0g
Cholesterol: 0mg
Sodium: 130mg
Total Carbohydrates: 46g
Dietary Fiber: 8g
Sugars: 23g
Protein: 20g
Vitamin D: 0%
Calcium: 20%
Iron: 6%
Potassium: 8%

5. Chia seed pudding with almond milk and fresh fruit

Ingredients:

- 1 cup of chia seeds
- 3 cups of almond milk

- 1 tsp of vanilla extract
- 2 tbsp of maple syrup or honey
- Fresh fruit of your choice for topping (e.g. berries, mango, kiwi, etc.)

Instructions:

- In a large bowl, mix together the chia seeds, almond milk, vanilla extract, and maple syrup or honey.
- Stir until well combined and the chia seeds have started to absorb the liquid.
- Cover the bowl with plastic wrap and let it sit in the fridge for at least 2 hours or overnight.
- Once the chia seeds have formed a gel-like texture, give the mixture a good stir and spoon it into serving glasses or bowls.
- Top with your favorite fresh fruit and enjoy!

Serving size: 4 servings

Nutritional value per serving:

Calories: 223
Fat: 12.9g
Carbohydrates: 22.3g
Protein: 8.3g
Fiber: 11.3g
Note: Nutritional values may vary depending on the type of almond milk and sweetener used.

6. Veggie and cheese frittata

Ingredients:

- 6 large eggs
- 1/2 cup of milk
- 1/4 cup of grated Parmesan cheese
- 1/4 teaspoon of salt
- 1/4 teaspoon of black pepper
- 1 tablespoon of olive oil
- 1 cup of diced onion
- 1 cup of diced bell pepper
- 1 cup of diced zucchini
- 1/2 cup of diced mushrooms

- 1 cup of shredded cheddar cheese

Instructions:

- In a large bowl, whisk together the eggs, milk, Parmesan cheese, salt, and pepper.

- In a large skillet, heat the olive oil over medium heat. Add the onion, bell pepper, zucchini, and mushrooms, and cook until they are soft, about 5 minutes.

- Pour the egg mixture into the skillet with the vegetables, and cook until the edges are set, about 5 minutes.

- Sprinkle the shredded cheddar cheese on top of the frittata, and cook until the cheese is melted, about 2 minutes.

- Slide the frittata onto a serving plate, and cut into slices. Serve immediately.

Serving Size: 6

Nutritional Value (per serving):

Calories: 236
Protein: 16 g
Fat: 18 g
Saturated Fat: 8 g
Carbohydrates: 8 g
Sugar: 3 g
Fiber: 2 g
Sodium: 464 mg
Cholesterol: 267 mg

7. Almond flour pancakes with almond butter and syrup

Ingredients:

- 1 and 1/2 cups almond flour
- 3 large eggs
- 1/4 cup almond milk
- 1 tsp vanilla extract
- 1 tsp baking powder

- 1/4 tsp salt
- 2 tbsp almond butter
- Maple syrup for serving

Instructions:

- In a medium bowl, whisk together the almond flour, eggs, almond milk, vanilla extract, baking powder, and salt.
- Heat a non-stick pan over medium heat.
- Use a 1/4 cup measure to pour batter onto the pan.
- Cook for 2-3 minutes on each side, or until lightly browned.
- Repeat with remaining batter.
- Serve pancakes with almond butter and maple syrup.

Nutritional Value per Pancake (with 2 tablespoons almond butter and 1 tablespoon maple syrup):

Calories: 300

Fat: 25g

Protein: 9g
Carbohydrates: 16g
Fiber: 3g
Serving size: 2 pancakes.

8. Turkey bacon and egg muffins

Ingredients:

- 8 slices of turkey bacon
- 8 large eggs
- 1/4 cup milk
- 1/4 tsp salt
- 1/4 tsp black pepper
- 1/4 cup shredded cheese (optional)
- Non-stick cooking spray

Instructions:

- Preheat the oven to 375°F (190°C).
- Line a muffin tin with 8 muffin cups and spray with non-stick cooking spray.

- Cut the turkey bacon into small pieces and cook until crispy in a pan on medium heat. Drain the excess fat.
- In a large bowl, beat the eggs, milk, salt, and black pepper together.
- Add the cooked bacon and cheese (if desired) to the egg mixture and stir to combine.
- Pour the egg mixture evenly into the muffin cups.
- Bake in the preheated oven for 18-20 minutes, or until the eggs are set.
- Let the muffins cool for a few minutes before removing them from the muffin tin.

Serving Size: 1 muffin

Nutritional Value (per serving):

Calories: 140
Fat: 10 g
Saturated Fat: 3 g
Cholesterol: 210 mg
Sodium: 470 mg

Carbohydrates: 1 g
Fiber: 0 g
Sugar: 1 g
Protein: 12 g

9. Cottage cheese with peaches and honey

Ingredients:

- 1 cup of cottage cheese
- 1 cup of peaches, diced
- 2 tbsp of honey

Nutritional value (per serving size):

Calories: 282
Fat: 7g
Saturated Fat: 4g
Cholesterol: 31mg
Sodium: 564 mg
Carbohydrates: 37g
Fiber: 2g
Sugar: 31g
Protein: 22g

Serving size: 1 cup

Instructions:

- In a bowl, mix the cottage cheese and peaches together.
- Drizzle honey over the mixture and stir well.
- Serve and enjoy your cottage cheese with peaches and honey!

10. Smoothie bowl with Greek yogurt, frozen berries, and almond milk.

Ingredients:

- 1 cup of frozen mixed berries (strawberries, blueberries, and raspberries)
- 1 cup of Greek yogurt
- 1 cup of almond milk
- 1 tablespoon of honey

- 1/2 teaspoon of vanilla extract
- 1 scoop of whey protein (optional)
- Toppings: granola, fresh berries, chia seeds, and almond slices

Instructions:

- Place the frozen berries, Greek yogurt, almond milk, honey, and vanilla extract in a blender.
- Blend until smooth and creamy.
- If using, add a scoop of whey protein and blend again until well combined.
- Pour the smoothie mixture into a bowl and add the desired toppings.
- Serve immediately and enjoy your healthy and delicious smoothie bowl.

Nutritional Information (per serving size of 1 bowl):

Calories: 365
Fat: 9.3 g
Saturated Fat: 2.3 g
Cholesterol: 17 mg
Sodium: 151 mg

Carbohydrates: 54.8 g
Fiber: 7.2 g
Sugar: 34.8 g
Protein: 22.2 g
Serving Size: 1 bowl (24 ounces)

Lunch Recipe

1. **Grilled chicken salad with mixed greens, cherry tomatoes, and avocado.**

Ingredients:

- 4 boneless, skinless chicken breasts
- 1 tsp. olive oil
- Salt and pepper, to taste
- 5 cups mixed greens
- 1 cup cherry tomatoes, halved
- 1 avocado, diced
- 2 tbsp. balsamic vinaigrette

Instructions:

- Preheat the grill to medium heat.
- Brush chicken with olive oil and sprinkle it with salt and pepper.
- Place chicken on the grill and cook for 5-7 minutes on each side, or until fully cooked.
- Remove chicken from the grill and let it cool for a few minutes.
- Slice chicken into strips.
- In a large bowl, combine mixed greens, cherry tomatoes, and avocado.
- Add sliced chicken and drizzle with balsamic vinaigrette. Toss to combine.
- Serve immediately.

Serving size: 4

Nutritional Value (per serving):
Calories: 326
Protein: 38 g
Fat: 17 g
Carbs: 13 g
Fiber: 6 g

Sugar: 5 g
Sodium: 302 mg

2. **Turkey, cheese, and lettuce wrap with salsa and guacamole.**

Ingredients:

- 4 large flour tortillas
- 4 ounces sliced turkey breast
- 4 slices of cheddar cheese
- 4 leaves of lettuce
- 1/2 cup salsa
- 1/2 cup guacamole

Instructions:

- Warm the flour tortillas in a microwave for 10-15 seconds or on a hot pan for a few seconds on each side.
- Place a slice of cheese on each tortilla.
- Add a few slices of turkey on top of the cheese.

- Place a lettuce leaf on top of the turkey.
- Spoon 1 tablespoon of salsa and 1 tablespoon of guacamole on each wrap.
- Fold the bottom and sides of the tortilla to create a wrap.
- Repeat the process for the remaining 3 wraps.

Serving size: 4 wraps

Nutritional value per wrap:

Calories: 371
Fat: 18 g
Saturated Fat: 6 g
Cholesterol: 42 mg
Sodium: 1051 mg
Carbohydrates: 33 g
Fiber: 3 g
Sugar: 3 g
Protein: 21 g

3. Veggie and egg scramble with spinach, bell peppers, onions, and mushrooms.

Ingredients:

- 1 tsp olive oil
- 1/2 cup chopped bell peppers
- 1/2 cup chopped onions
- 1/2 cup chopped mushrooms
- 2 cups fresh spinach
- 4 eggs
- Salt and pepper to taste

Instructions:

- Heat a large non-stick pan over medium heat. Add the olive oil and swirl to coat the pan.

- Add the chopped bell peppers, onions, and mushrooms. Sauté until the vegetables are tender, about 5-7 minutes.

- Add the fresh spinach to the pan and stir until wilted, about 2 minutes.

- In a separate bowl, beat the eggs with salt and pepper to taste.

- Pour the beaten eggs into the pan and scramble until fully cooked, about 3-5 minutes.

- Serve the veggie and egg scramble hot, garnished with additional salt and pepper if desired.

Serving Size: 4 portions

Nutritional Value (per serving):

Calories: 150
Fat: 10g
Protein: 11g
Carbohydrates: 8g
Fiber: 2g
Sodium: 80mg

4. **Tuna salad with celery, pickles, and mayonnaise on whole grain bread.**

Serving size: 1 sandwich

Ingredients:

- 2 ounces canned tuna, drained
- 2 tablespoons diced celery
- 2 tablespoons diced pickles
- 2 tablespoons mayonnaise
- 2 slices of whole grain bread
- Salt and pepper, to taste

Instructions:

- In a medium bowl, mix the canned tuna, celery, pickles, mayonnaise, salt and pepper.
- Toast the slices of whole grain bread.
- Spread the tuna mixture evenly on one slice of the toasted bread.

- Top with the other slice of toasted bread.
- Serve immediately.

Nutritional Value per Serving:

Calories: 350
Fat: 18g
Saturated Fat: 2g
Cholesterol: 25mg
Sodium: 500mg
Carbohydrates: 33g
Fiber: 7g
Sugar: 4g
Protein: 17g

5. Grilled salmon with roasted vegetables and quinoa.

Ingredients:

- 4 salmon filets, 6 oz each
- 1 large sweet potato, peeled and diced
- 2 red bell peppers, sliced
- 1 large red onion, sliced
- 2 tablespoons olive oil

- Salt and pepper, to taste
- 1 cup quinoa, rinsed
- 2 cups chicken broth
- 1 tablespoon lemon juice

Instructions:

- Preheat the oven to 400°F.

- In a large mixing bowl, combine the diced sweet potato, sliced red bell peppers, and sliced red onion. Add 2 tablespoons of olive oil and season with salt and pepper to taste.

- Transfer the vegetables to a roasting pan and roast in the oven for 25-30 minutes or until tender.

- While the vegetables are roasting, rinse the quinoa in a fine mesh strainer.

- In a saucepan, bring 2 cups of chicken broth to a boil. Stir in the rinsed quinoa and reduce the heat to low. Cover the saucepan with a lid and cook for 18-20 minutes or until the quinoa is tender and the liquid has been absorbed.

- Preheat the grill to medium-high heat.

- Season the salmon filets with salt and pepper to taste. Place the salmon filets on the grill and cook for 6-7 minutes per side or until the salmon is cooked through.
- L
- In a small bowl, whisk together 1 tablespoon of lemon juice with a pinch of salt and pepper. Drizzle the lemon juice over the cooked quinoa and fluff with a fork to mix well.

- To serve, divide the cooked quinoa between 4 serving plates. Top each plate with a salmon filet and a serving of the roasted vegetables.

Serving Size: 4 portions, 6 oz salmon filet, 1 cup quinoa, and 1 serving of roasted vegetables.

Nutritional Value (per serving):

Calories: 560
Fat: 22g
Saturated Fat: 3g
Cholesterol: 94mg
Sodium: 474mg
Carbohydrates: 49g
Fiber: 7g
Sugar: 7g
Protein: 39g

6. Greek yogurt with mixed berries, almonds, and a drizzle of honey.

Ingredients:

- 1 cup Greek yogurt

- 1/2 cup mixed berries (strawberries, blueberries, raspberries)
- 1/4 cup almonds, chopped
- 1 tbsp honey

Instructions:

- In a bowl, add the Greek yogurt.
- Wash and chop the mixed berries and add them on top of the yogurt.
- Sprinkle the chopped almonds on top of the berries.
- Drizzle the honey over the almonds and berries.
- Serve and enjoy!

Nutritional Information:

Serves 1
Total calories: 330
Fat: 17g
Cholesterol: 10mg
Sodium: 170mg
Total carbohydrates: 33g
Dietary fiber: 4g
Sugars: 22g

Protein: 18g

7. Broiled shrimp skewers with cucumber and tomato salad.

Ingredients:

- 1 lb. raw large shrimp, peeled and deveined
- 1 tbsp. olive oil
- 1 tsp. lemon juice
- 1 tsp. paprika
- 1 tsp. garlic powder
- Salt and pepper to taste
- 2 medium cucumbers, peeled and sliced
- 2 medium tomatoes, sliced
- 2 tbsp. red wine vinegar
- 2 tbsp. olive oil
- 1 tsp. honey
- Salt and pepper to taste

Instructions:

- Preheat the broiler to high heat.

- In a large bowl, combine the shrimp, olive oil, lemon juice, paprika, garlic powder, salt and pepper. Stir until the shrimp are evenly coated.

- Thread the shrimp on skewers. Place the skewers on a broiling pan and broil for 4-5 minutes per side or until the shrimp are pink and opaque.

- Meanwhile, in another large bowl, combine the cucumbers, tomatoes, red wine vinegar, olive oil, honey, salt and pepper. Toss until the vegetables are evenly coated.

- Serve the broiled shrimp skewers with the cucumber and tomato salad on the side.

Serving size: 4

Nutritional value per serving:

Calories: 250

Fat: 18 g

Saturated Fat: 2 g

Cholesterol: 145 mg

Sodium: 420 mg

Carbohydrates: 9 g

Fiber: 2 g

Protein: 16 g

8. Veggie and hummus wrap with carrots, bell peppers, and red onions.

Ingredients:

- 4 large flour tortillas
- 1 cup hummus
- 2 medium carrots, sliced
- 1 red bell pepper, sliced
- 1/2 red onion, sliced
- Salt and pepper to taste

Serving size: 4 wraps

Instructions:

- Spread 1/4 cup of hummus on each tortilla.
- Place the sliced carrots, bell pepper, and red onion in a row on top of the hummus.
- Season with salt and pepper to taste.
- Roll the tortilla tightly, tucking in the ends to secure the fillings.
- Repeat with the remaining tortillas.
- Slice each wrap in half and serve.

Nutritional Value:

Each wrap contains approximately:
250 calories

10g of protein
36g of carbohydrates
9g of fat
7g of fiber
350mg of sodium.

9. Peanut butter and banana sandwich on whole grain bread.

Ingredients:
- 2 slices of whole grain bread
- 2 tablespoons of creamy peanut butter
- 1 medium-sized ripe banana, sliced

Nutritional Value (per serving):
Calories: 460
Fat: 24g
Saturated Fat: 4g
Cholesterol: 0mg
Sodium: 480mg
Carbohydrates: 53g
Fiber: 10g

Sugar: 15g
Protein: 16g

Serving size: 1 sandwich (2 slices)

Instructions:

- Toast the two slices of whole grain bread to your desired level of crispiness.
- Spread 1 tablespoon of creamy peanut butter on each slice of bread.
- Place sliced banana on one slice of bread and close the sandwich with the other slice.
- Cut the sandwich in half and serve.
- Enjoy this classic and delicious sandwich that is high in protein and fiber, making it a great option for a filling and nutritious breakfast or snack.

10. Lentil soup with mixed greens and a side of whole grain crackers.

Ingredients:

- 2 cups green lentils
- 1 onion, chopped
- 2 cloves garlic, minced
- 2 tablespoons olive oil
- 1 teaspoon dried thyme
- 4 cups vegetable broth
- 4 cups water
- 1 cup mixed greens (kale, spinach, Swiss chard, etc.)
- Salt and pepper to taste
- 8 whole grain crackers

Instructions:

- In a large pot, heat the olive oil over medium heat. Add the onion and cook until soft and translucent, about 5 minutes.

- Add the garlic and thyme and cook for another minute.

- Add the lentils, vegetable broth, and water to the pot and bring to a boil.

- Reduce heat to low and let the soup simmer for about 30 minutes, or until the lentils are tender.

- Stir in the mixed greens and cook until wilted, about 5 minutes.

- Season with salt and pepper to taste.

- Serve the soup with whole grain crackers on the side.

Serving Size: 4

Nutritional Value:

Per serving, the lentil soup provides approximately:

480 calories

20g of protein

64g of carbohydrates

14g of fat

12g of fiber

7g of sugar

This lentil soup is a filling and nutritious meal that provides a good source of protein, fiber, and vitamins from the mixed greens. The whole grain crackers add an extra crunch and some whole grains to the meal.

Dinner Recipe

1. Grilled Chicken Salad with Avocado Dressing

Ingredients:

- 4 boneless, skinless chicken breasts
- Salt and pepper
- 1 large head of lettuce, chopped
- 2 medium avocados

- 1/4 cup plain Greek yogurt
- 2 tablespoons freshly squeezed lemon juice
- 2 tablespoons olive oil
- 2 cloves of garlic, minced
- 1/4 teaspoon salt
- 1/4 teaspoon black pepper
- 1/2 red onion, thinly sliced
- 1 cup cherry tomatoes, halved
- 1/2 cup crumbled feta cheese

Instructions:

- Preheat the grill to medium-high heat.
- Season the chicken breasts with salt and pepper on both sides.
- Place the chicken on the grill and cook for 6-8 minutes on each side, or until fully cooked through.
- Remove from heat and let cool for 5 minutes.
- Cut the chicken into thin slices.
- In a blender, combine the avocados, Greek yogurt, lemon juice, olive oil,

garlic, salt, and pepper. Blend until smooth.

- In a large bowl, add the chopped lettuce, red onion, cherry tomatoes, sliced chicken, and crumbled feta cheese.
- Toss the ingredients with the avocado dressing.
- Serve immediately.

Serving size: 4

Nutritional value per serving:

Calories: 448
Fat: 33 g
Saturated fat: 8 g
Cholesterol: 66 mg
Sodium: 536 mg
Carbohydrates: 17 g
Fiber: 8 g
Sugar: 5 g
Protein: 27 g

2. Broiled Salmon with Roasted Vegetables

Ingredients:

- 4 salmon filets (6 oz each)
- 1 large zucchini, sliced
- 1 large yellow squash, sliced
- 1 red bell pepper, sliced
- 1 yellow onion, sliced
- 4 cloves of garlic, minced
- 1 tbsp olive oil
- Salt and pepper to taste
- Lemon wedges (optional)

Instructions:

- Preheat the oven to 400°F.
- Line a large baking sheet with parchment paper.
- Arrange the sliced zucchini, yellow squash, red bell pepper, and onion on the prepared baking sheet.

- Drizzle olive oil over the vegetables and sprinkle with salt, pepper, and minced garlic. Toss to combine.
- Roast the vegetables for 25-30 minutes, or until tender and slightly charred.
- Meanwhile, season the salmon filets with salt and pepper.
- Place the salmon filets on a separate baking sheet and broil for 8-10 minutes, or until the skin is crispy and the salmon is cooked through.
- Serve the broiled salmon with the roasted vegetables on the side, and lemon wedges if desired.

Serving size: 4 servings (1 salmon filet and 1 cup of roasted vegetables per serving)

Nutritional Information (per serving):

Calories: 350
Fat: 20 g
Saturated Fat: 3 g
Cholesterol: 107 mg

Sodium: 227 mg
Carbohydrates: 10 g
Fiber: 3 g
Protein: 34 g

3. Veggie Stir-Fry with Tofu and Brown Rice

Ingredients:

- 1 package of extra-firm tofu, cubed
- 1 cup of mixed vegetables (such as broccoli, bell peppers, carrots, and mushrooms)
- 1 tablespoon of canola oil
- 1 tablespoon of soy sauce
- 1 teaspoon of cornstarch
- 2 cups of cooked brown rice

Instructions:

- Press the tofu between paper towels to remove excess water.
- In a wok or large pan, heat the canola oil over medium-high heat. Add the

tofu and stir-fry for 5-7 minutes until browned.
- Add the mixed vegetables to the pan and stir-fry for another 5 minutes until tender.
- In a small bowl, mix the soy sauce and cornstarch. Add the mixture to the pan and stir until the sauce has thickened.
- Serve the stir-fry over the cooked brown rice.

Serving Size: 2

Nutritional Value (per serving):

Calories: 430
Fat: 16g
Saturated Fat: 2g
Cholesterol: 0mg
Sodium: 900mg
Carbohydrates: 57g
Fiber: 7g
Protein: 21g

4. Turkey Chili with Beans and Sweet Potatoes

Ingredients:

- 1 lb. ground turkey
- 1 large onion, chopped
- 2 cloves garlic, minced
- 1 red bell pepper, chopped
- 1 green bell pepper, chopped
- 2 medium sweet potatoes, peeled and diced
- 1 can black beans, drained and rinsed
- 1 can kidney beans, drained and rinsed
- 1 can diced tomatoes
- 2 tbsp. chili powder
- 1 tsp. ground cumin
- 1 tsp. dried oregano
- 1 tsp. salt
- 1/2 tsp. black pepper
- 2 cups chicken broth

Instructions:

- Heat a large pot over medium heat and add the ground turkey. Cook until browned, breaking it up into small pieces as it cooks.
- Add the chopped onion, minced garlic, chopped red and green bell peppers, and diced sweet potatoes to the pot and cook for 5-7 minutes, until the vegetables are slightly softened.
- Add the drained and rinsed black and kidney beans, diced tomatoes, chili powder, cumin, oregano, salt, and black pepper to the pot. Stir to combine.
- Pour in the chicken broth and bring the chili to a boil. Reduce heat to low and let it simmer for 20-30 minutes, until the sweet potatoes are tender and the flavors have had a chance to develop.
- Serve hot with your favorite toppings such as shredded cheese, sour cream, and chopped cilantro.

Serving size: 6

Nutritional Value (per serving):
Calories: 298
Total Fat: 8g
Saturated Fat: 2g
Cholesterol: 75mg
Sodium: 738 mg
Total Carbohydrates: 33g
Dietary Fiber: 9g
Sugars: 8g
Protein: 26g

5. Baked Eggplant Parmesan with Whole Wheat Pasta

Ingredients:

- 2 medium sized eggplants, sliced
- 1 cup all-purpose flour
- 2 eggs, beaten
- 1 cup seasoned bread crumbs
- 1 cup marinara sauce
- 1 cup shredded mozzarella cheese
- 1/4 cup grated parmesan cheese

- Salt and pepper, to taste
- 8 oz whole wheat pasta
- Fresh basil leaves, for garnish (optional)

Instructions:

- Preheat the oven to 375°F (190°C). Line a baking sheet with parchment paper.
- Place the flour in a shallow dish and season with salt and pepper.
- In another shallow dish, beat the eggs.
- In a third shallow dish, mix the breadcrumbs, parmesan cheese, and salt and pepper.
- Dip each eggplant slice in the flour, then the eggs, and finally the breadcrumb mixture. Place the coated eggplant slices on the prepared baking sheet.
- Bake the eggplant slices for 15 minutes, or until they are crispy and golden brown.

- Meanwhile, cook the pasta according to the package instructions. Drain and set aside.
- In a large oven-proof dish, spread a layer of marinara sauce on the bottom. Top with a layer of eggplant slices and a sprinkle of mozzarella cheese. Repeat until all ingredients are used, ending with a layer of mozzarella cheese.
- Bake the eggplant parmesan for 15 minutes, or until the cheese is melted and bubbly.
- Serve the eggplant parmesan over the whole wheat pasta. Garnish with fresh basil leaves, if desired.

Serving size: 4 servings

Nutritional Information per serving:

Calories: 410
Total Fat: 14 g
Saturated Fat: 5 g
Cholesterol: 97 mg

Sodium: 578 mg
Total Carbohydrates: 55 g
Dietary Fiber: 9 g
Sugars: 10 g
Protein: 19 g

6. Spaghetti Squash with Turkey Meat Sauce

Ingredients:

- 1 medium spaghetti squash
- 1 lb. ground turkey
- 1 large onion, chopped
- 3 garlic cloves, minced
- 1 can (28 oz) of crushed tomatoes
- 2 tbsp tomato paste
- 2 tbsp dried basil
- 1 tsp dried oregano
- 1 tsp dried thyme
- Salt and pepper to taste
- 2 tbsp olive oil

- Fresh grated parmesan cheese for serving (optional)

Instructions:

- Preheat the oven to 400°F.
- Cut the spaghetti squash in half lengthwise and remove the seeds.
- Place the two halves cut-side down on a baking sheet lined with parchment paper.
- Bake for 25-30 minutes, or until the squash is tender.
- In a large skillet, heat the olive oil over medium heat.
- Add the chopped onion and minced garlic and cook until softened, about 5 minutes.
- Add the ground turkey to the skillet and cook until browned, breaking up any large chunks.
- Stir in the crushed tomatoes, tomato paste, dried basil, oregano, thyme, salt, and pepper.

- Reduce heat to low and let the sauce simmer for 15-20 minutes.
- Use a fork to gently scrape the spaghetti squash flesh into long strands.
- Serve the spaghetti squash topped with the turkey meat sauce and grated parmesan cheese.

Serving Size: 4

Nutritional Value (per serving):

Calories: 325
Fat: 14 g
Saturated Fat: 3 g
Cholesterol: 81 mg
Sodium: 517 mg
Carbohydrates: 27 g
Fiber: 5 g
Sugar: 10 g
Protein: 27 g

7. Quinoa and Black Bean Bowl with Salsa and Guacamole

Ingredients:

- 1 cup quinoa
- 1 can black beans, drained and rinsed
- 1 cup salsa
- 1 avocado, mashed
- 2 tablespoons lime juice
- Salt and pepper to taste
- Optional toppings: shredded cheese, sour cream, cilantro

Serving size: 4 bowls

Instructions:

- Rinse the quinoa in a fine mesh strainer and add to a pot with 2 cups of water. Bring to a boil, then reduce heat to low and simmer for 15-20 minutes, or until the quinoa is tender and the water has been absorbed.

- In a separate bowl, mix the mashed avocado with the lime juice, salt, and pepper to make the guacamole.
- In each bowl, add 1/4 cup of cooked quinoa and 1/4 cup of black beans.
- Top each bowl with 1/4 cup of salsa and a spoonful of guacamole.
- Add any additional toppings, if desired.

Nutrition per serving:

Cal: 368
Fat: 14g
Carbs: 56g
Protein: 14g
Fiber: 12g

8. Lentil and Vegetable Soup with Whole Wheat Croutons

Ingredients:

- 1 cup dried green lentils
- 4 cups vegetable broth

- 2 tablespoons olive oil
- 1 onion, chopped
- 3 carrots, chopped
- 3 celery stalks, chopped
- 4 cloves garlic, minced
- 1 teaspoon dried thyme
- 1 teaspoon dried basil
- 1 teaspoon dried oregano
- 2 large tomatoes, chopped
- 4 cups chopped kale
- 2 cups cubed whole wheat bread

Instructions:

1. Rinse the lentils and place them in a large pot. Add the vegetable broth and bring to a boil. Reduce heat and let simmer for 25-30 minutes, or until lentils are tender.

2. In a large pan, heat the olive oil over medium heat. Add the onion, carrots, celery, and garlic and cook until vegetables are soft, about 5 minutes.

3. Stir in the thyme, basil, oregano, and chopped tomatoes. Add the vegetable mixture to the lentil pot and continue to simmer for 10-15 minutes.

4. Stir in the chopped kale and let it cook for another 5 minutes, or until it is wilted.

5. Preheat the oven to 400°F. Place the cubed whole wheat bread on a baking sheet and bake for 10-12 minutes, or until they are crispy and golden brown.

6. Serve the lentil soup with the whole wheat croutons.

Serving Size: 8 servings

Nutritional Value per serving:

Calories: 236
Protein: 12g

Fat: 7g
Carbohydrates: 34g
Fiber: 9g
Sugar: 5g
Sodium: 630mg

9. Grilled Pork Tenderloin with Roasted Carrots and Sweet Potatoes

Ingredients:

- 2 pounds pork tenderloin
- 2 pounds carrots, sliced
- 2 pounds sweet potatoes, peeled and diced
- 2 tablespoons olive oil
- 1 teaspoon dried thyme
- Salt and pepper to taste

Instructions:

- Preheat the grill to medium-high heat.

- In a mixing bowl, combine olive oil, thyme, salt, and pepper.
- Rub the pork tenderloin with the mixture, making sure it is evenly coated.
- Place the pork tenderloin on the grill and cook for about 10-15 minutes on each side or until the internal temperature reaches 145°F.
- While the pork is cooking, preheat the oven to 400°F.
- In a large mixing bowl, combine sliced carrots and diced sweet potatoes with 2 tablespoons of olive oil, salt, and pepper.
- Spread the mixture in a single layer on a baking sheet and roast for 25-30 minutes or until tender and slightly golden.
- Serve the grilled pork tenderloin with roasted carrots and sweet potatoes.

Serving Size: 4

Nutritional Value (per serving):

Calories: 647
Fat: 20g
Carbohydrates: 54g
Protein: 64g
Fiber: 9g

Note: The nutritional value may vary depending on the brand and type of ingredients used.

10. Vegetable and Tuna Salad with Balsamic Vinegar Dressing

Ingredients:

- 2 heads of lettuce, chopped
- 1 medium carrot, grated
- 1 medium cucumber, sliced
- 1 medium tomato, chopped
- 1 medium red onion, sliced
- 2 cans of tuna, drained and flaked
- 1/4 cup of balsamic vinegar

- 2 tablespoons of extra-virgin olive oil
- 1 teaspoon of Dijon mustard
- Salt and pepper to taste

Instructions:

- In a large bowl, combine the lettuce, carrot, cucumber, tomato, and red onion.
- Add the flaked tuna and mix well.
- In a small bowl, whisk together the balsamic vinegar, olive oil, Dijon mustard, salt, and pepper.
- Pour the dressing over the salad and toss to coat evenly.
- Serve immediately.

Serving Size: 4

Nutritional Value:

Calories: 250
Fat: 15g
Saturated Fat: 2g
Cholesterol: 40mg
Sodium: 480mg

Carbohydrates: 11g
Fiber: 3g
Sugar: 6g
Protein: 19g

Chapter 6

Maintenance and Sustainability

Staying Committed to Intermittent Fasting

It might be difficult for women over 40 to remain dedicated to intermittent fasting. Here are some pointers to keep you motivated to maintain this way of life:

Prior to beginning your intermittent fasting adventure, make definite, attainable objectives. Keep a list of your goals, including things like weight reduction, better digestion, and more mental clarity, close to hand.

Make a sensible plan first since intermittent fasting is not a one-size-fits-all strategy. Start with a schedule that works for you, such as 16 hours of fasting followed by 8 hours of eating. Increase the fasting time gradually as your body gets used to it.

Keep your body hydrated by drinking plenty of water during any fasting times. Additionally, this will aid in setting your appetite.

Eat nutrient-dense foods throughout your eating intervals and don't miss meals. It will be challenging to maintain your fasting schedule if you skip meals since doing so will simply make you feel hungry and exhausted.

Join a support group to share your experiences and get encouragement. Examples of such groups include online communities and fitness classes. Additionally, it helps keep you responsible and inspired.

Be aware while eating since intermittent fasting involves more than simply what you consume. Utilize mindfulness when eating by taking your time and appreciating each mouthful. You'll feel more full of yourself and eat less as a result.

Though intermittent fasting isn't always simple, it's crucial to remain upbeat and remind yourself of its advantages. Don't punish yourself if you make a mistake. Get back on course and continue to be dedicated to your objectives.

You may enjoy the numerous advantages of intermittent fasting and keep up a healthy lifestyle as a woman over 40 by adhering to these suggestions and being dedicated.

Implementing Intermittent Fasting in Your Life

A form of eating pattern known as intermittent fasting involves alternating between periods of fasting and eating. The various health advantages of this eating strategy, such as weight reduction, an enhanced metabolism, and a lower risk of chronic illnesses, have helped it gain popularity in recent years.

However, many women over the age of 40 would question if this kind of eating habit is suitable for them and their fluctuating hormone levels. The good news is that intermittent fasting may still be beneficial for women over 40. Here are some suggestions to help you incorporate it into your life:

Start Slowly: It's advised to begin intermittent fasting slowly and gradually if you're a beginner. Start with a 12-hour fast, then progressively extend it until you achieve your ideal fasting length.

The 16/8 approach, the 5:2 diet, and alternate-day fasting are just a few of the many intermittent fasting strategies available. Pick the one that best suits your lifestyle and schedule.

Keep Hydrated: To prevent dehydration when fasting, be sure to consume lots of water. Additionally, you may sip on unsweetened tea or coffee.

Consume a Healthy Diet: Intermittent fasting is not a justification for eating junk food. Eat a healthy, balanced diet that is high in fresh produce, whole grains, lean protein, and other nutrients.

Take Note of Your Body: Pay close attention to how your body reacts to the modifications to your food schedule. Adjust your fasting schedule to include extra eating times if you're feeling fatigued or having problems focusing.

Be Consistent: Intermittent fasting works best when a regular schedule is followed. On the same days each week, try to fast and eat.

Keep Moving: Whether or whether you engage in intermittent fasting, exercise is crucial to maintaining a healthy lifestyle. To boost your general health and wellbeing, be sure to engage in a lot of physical exercise.

In conclusion, women over 40 may still benefit from intermittent fasting if they start out slowly, choose the appropriate fasting technique, keep hydrated, eat a good diet, pay attention to their bodies, are consistent, and maintain an active lifestyle. Before beginning any new food or fitness routine, remember to check with your doctor to be sure it is suitable for your particular health requirements.

Preventing Plateaus and Relapses

The body's metabolism might slow down as a woman ages, making it more challenging to lose weight and keep it off. It's crucial to know how to avoid plateaus and relapses while using intermittent fasting as a weight reduction method.

Avoid Restrictive Fasting: Before beginning an intermittent fasting regimen, it's crucial to steer clear of going extended periods without eating or drinking. This may result in a slowed metabolism, which will make weight loss more challenging. Instead, try to keep your fasts shorter, like 16 hours without eating, followed by 8 hours.

Increase Your Exercise: Exercise might help you burn more calories and avoid plateaus. Aim for 30 minutes of daily, moderate activity, like cycling or walking. Additionally helpful for gaining muscle and boosting metabolism, resistance exercise.

Maintaining a regular schedule of exercise and intermittent fasting is essential for avoiding plateaus and relapses. Avoid missing your fasting days or skipping your workouts.

Maintaining a healthy metabolism and avoiding plateaus need enough hydration. Aim for eight glasses of water or more each day.

Track Progress: Monitoring your development may help you see possible roadblocks that might result in plateaus and relapses. To keep tabs on your diet, workout routine, and weight, keep a food journal.

Change Up Your Routine: Keeping things fresh will help you stay motivated and avoid plateaus. Try varying your fasting times, stepping up the level of your workout, or trying something new.

Stay away from processed foods since they are heavy in calories, bad fats, and added sugars. Avoiding these foods may assist in maintaining weight reduction and preventing relapses.

In conclusion, maintaining consistency, exercising, staying hydrated, monitoring progress, switching up routines, and avoiding processed meals are all necessary to prevent plateaus and relapses in intermittent fasting for women over 40. You may effectively sustain weight reduction and meet your health and fitness goals by heeding the advice in this article.

.

Conclusion

The Power of Intermittent Fasting for Women Over 40

Recent years have seen a lot of interest in the popular diet trend known as intermittent fasting. In order to reduce calorie consumption and encourage weight reduction, this diet alternates between eating and fasting times. Many individuals have been proven to benefit from it, although women over 40 benefit the most.

Hormone regulation is one of the key advantages of intermittent fasting for women over 40. The hormonal imbalance that occurs as women age may lead to weight gain, mood changes, and other health issues. Women may assist manage their hormones and maintain a healthy balance by managing when and what they consume.

Additionally, intermittent fasting enhances metabolism, which facilitates weight loss in women over 40. This is so that dangerous poisons and waste materials may be eliminated from the body by activating cellular cleansing activities during fasting times. This enhances the body's general performance, which results in more energy and weight reduction.

Intermittent fasting has additional advantages for women over 40 since it may lower their chance of developing chronic illnesses like diabetes and heart disease. This is due to the diet's ability to control blood sugar levels and lower inflammation, both of which may aid in delaying the onset of these illnesses.

Finally, because women over 40 may select when to fast and when to eat based on their schedules and lifestyles, intermittent fasting may be a practical and adaptable diet choice for them. Because of this, they may simply adopt the diet without having to make significant lifestyle adjustments.

In conclusion, intermittent fasting may be a potent tool for women over 40, assisting in hormone regulation, enhancing metabolism, lowering the risk of chronic illnesses, and being a practical and adaptable diet alternative. As with any diet, it's crucial to see a healthcare practitioner to make sure it's safe and suited to each person's requirements before beginning.

www.ingramcontent.com/pod-product-compliance
Lightning Source LLC
Chambersburg PA
CBHW071022250726

48653CB00005B/1680